BIODYNAMICS OF OSTEOPATHY

Pediatrics Three

Second Edition

James Jealous D.O.

For more information about Dr. Jealous please visit:
https://BiodynamicsOfOsteopathy.com

BIODYNAMICS OF OSTEOPATHY Pediatrics Three

Hardback ISBN: 979-8-2955-3938-1

Second Edition 2025

James Jealous D.O. (1943–2021) practiced as an osteopathic physician, teacher and writer for many years. His life's work was to found and develop the specific methodology of Biodynamics of Osteopathy, following the lineage of Dr. A.T. Still and Dr. W.G. Sutherland.

This is one of a series of Biodynamics of Osteopathy books. They grew organically from sets of handouts written by Dr. Jealous and given to students during courses taught by him and his teachers. After many years he collected the handouts together and created individual course manuals, which he added to and rewrote many times. After several more years they evolved further into books.

TABLE OF CONTENTS

OSTEOPATHY IS SERVICE

We use our hands ...

To treat the Whole patient

To listen to the indwelling movements of Life

To treat all levels of illness

To assist in building the patient's functional reserve

To support homeostasis and trophicity by balancing the activity of the autonomic nervous system

To explore "laws not framed by human hands" (Dr. Still and Dr. Sutherland)

To cooperate and communicate with the Laws of Nature (Dr. Wales)

"To find the Health" (Dr. Still)

To get to the treatment plan

To get to the diagnosis

To help establish a point of Rest or Neutral around which the Whole can come to balance

To find Cause

We believe ...

We have an innate capacity to heal
The patient functions as a whole
The autonomic nervous system plays a major role in disease and healing
Structure and function are one form of activity
The Divine is indwelling
Life moves beyond death
There is a Constant Movement toward Normal
We are here to Serve Humanity

Normal is ...

"A sense of peace and harmony" (Dr. Sutherland)
Ease of motion, without tension
A capacity for Neutral
A sense of Wholeness to Life
The capacity for adaptation, change without compensation.

"Skill is proportionate to one's understanding of normal" (Dr. Still)

PERCEPTUAL STUDIES: THE FLOW OF THE ATTENTION

Motion is the essence of Life.
Where there is motion there is a natural flow of Neutrality and Wholeness.
Voluntary motion is controlled by the attention of the individual.
Involuntary motion is the expression of Wholeness.
Involuntary motion is the essence of osteopathy.
The flow of attention from the Seer creates the seen and the unseen.

***

Our attention can be quite fixed; that is, it lacks motion.
The state of our attention conditions what we perceive.
It also has a tremendous effect on our sense of wellness.
Stasis precedes disease.
Both disease and pain are related to static attention.
Education trains the attention to converge, to go to a place and hold there, stopping the natural flow and creating a separation from the Health. The result is loneliness and grief, often unseen, but lurking in the subconscious.
Normal attention flows like warm honey.
When it flows it is moved by the Health toward its cause.
We will study the flow/stasis of attention and observe the movement of the attention when it is free and flowing.
This task requires mental concentration.

THE STUDY OF THE ACTIVITY OF ATTENTION

"Our skill is proportionate to our understanding of normal."

Dr. Still's words will challenge us to look not at our capacity to find lesions but our ability to understand normal physiological motions. This knowledge is not in books. One must see normal by the power of observation.

What is the normal movement of attention?

We begin our study by watching our attention ...

Is it focused and fixed on a place?

Where is the fulcrum that controls the attention?

What is the cause of the act of attention?

Is it flowing from inside to outside ... freely ... fixed ... where does it originate ... all this we do by sensing the attention, as it works or as it locks up and lesions (stops flowing).

Let it flow to the interior of yourself. What does it do? Where does it flow? Does it stop on a thought or a feeling?

Does it flow into a place?

As the day passes, every once in a while, try to see what your attention is doing, and record the event ... remember, we are trying to understand normal; that is, what does the attention do when allowed to express its truth, its motion?

The attention is a substance, an energy that flows from the Source of Life, and as such it is naturally at "work," following the intention of the Breath of Life.

When the attention is free to move, one does not feel time, or death, or separation from anything, even enemies.

Ruby Day talked about attention as force. She said that Sutherland taught that it was more than enough force to add to a treatment when using midline dynamics. She trained me to know when to use the attention as a tool and when to literally withdraw it so it was not an inhibitory force. The attention was never fixed for more than a few seconds, and only in an attempt to ignite the reciprocal tension potency and set it in therapeutic motion, similar to a lateral fluctuation.

When someone fixes their attention too long, not only is it uncomfortable for the patient, but it can lesion living substances. The attention and the intention should flow through everything and not be directed by us … The flow of wisdom will do work that will organize everything into the flow of normal.

A neutral mind has no personal intention. It is impartial, lacks partiality to all things or outcomes, thus allowing the automatic shifting of one's perception by the River of Life.

It flows into the Meeting Place and the River of Life.

AN APPEAL TO THE THINKING OSTEOPATHS OF THE PROFESSION

Shall we permit the Osteopathic profession to be enslaved to the medical trust? ... As the father of the profession, I am making an international call ... I unfurled the Osteopathic flag of freedom over forty years ago ... Do not allow it to be trampled at the feet of our enemy. ... Osteopathy is yet in its infancy. I have only brought forth the principles and truth, which I have turned over to the profession, which has the wisdom and enough moral backbone not to offer any compromise ... IF we cannot have the pure Osteopathic principles taught in our schools, I hope ... we will build an international school that will offer no compromise ...

A. T. Still

Quoted from a letter by Dr. Andrew Taylor Still addressed to the president of the American Osteopathic Association in 1915. Printed in the 1948 A.O.A Yearbook.

INTRODUCTION

The principles of osteopathy emerged with Dr. Still and have unfolded in the hands of courageous men and women worldwide, since he observed natural laws at work in his patients and the world around him. Physicians who followed him had to swim against the currents of organized allopathic medicine and their own inner tendencies to think "against" lesions and not listen to the Wholeness of the Health.

The battle between the internal mind, mesmerized by finding lesions, and the deeper realities of observing indwelling therapeutic forces and the Health, is in fact a story that separates the traditional osteopaths from the more bland allopathic osteopathic thinkers.

If you understand what I mean, you are also aware that this mental orientation toward the deeper realities under your hands takes discipline and knowledge, and demands changing yourself in order to understand the depths of Still's philosophy and practice... this change suffuses all aspects of life, not just practice ... it is an awakening to the "voice" of our own Health.

This journey we take toward being a complete, uncompromised osteopath never ends, but the landscapes we traverse are full of beauty and majesty... one landscape is the dynamic world of children and their unfoldment. To get to this geography, one travels through a variety of terrains, each one unique and self-sustaining ... our task is to understand healing in the context of the whole patient and their interface with life, not our doctrinal overlays ... to see nature's wisdom one must be still... synchronize with her creative breath, and move in tempo with her intentions as they occur ... moment to moment, in a direction of ease.

The tools we need are "built in" but buried in our subconscious mind, remote from our daily habits. Being still is not easy for the educated mind, which is molded and synapsed by the environment of modern societies ... we actually learn not to listen but to react internally to the words we hear, as if we were always comparing our knowledge with what we hear rather than listening more completely on behalf of the speaker, be it a patient, Mother Nature, or the Divine ... children uncloaked by tedious "standards" approach life looking for the new ... for something not seen before ... something fresh. As adults we superimpose theories on the movements of life, unsuspecting that we are blind and deaf to most of reality.

Being stilled by the radiance of a child is beauty acting on us, to center us.

As we are transformed by this Health, we become synchronized with the breathing through everything ... a sweetness rarely found in oneself.

This unveils a new consciousness.

Then the tempo of the movement of the healing process becomes evident.

This is essential for the treatment of children in their terms, rather than correction of palpable restrictions. These principles allow one to meet the science of unfoldment that children experience, rather than an adult model of biomechanical lesions.

The science of unfoldment is called embryology. The mysterious force behind unfoldment is biodynamic (see Blechschmidt) or, as we call it, Primary Respiration (see Sutherland). These two sciences have a common seed from which they sprout ... this movement of unfoldment is the primary interest of this text.

How do children grow ... how do they heal ... this is our research and interest.

As we explore, we must, of necessity, challenge the biomechanical model, not with malice but for the purpose of science and clarity, realizing that one must shed the old skin in oneself in order to feel the new. Children are explorers by nature ... shedding and reforming as they go into the landscape of life ... they lean into the new, rather than withdraw ... Sutherland/Blechschmidt/ Still all had this calm pursuit of Wholeness ... it is within this framework that this writing moves forward.

The clinical results will prove to you that the changes you make are worth it.

INFUSED CENTERING

Doctor Still wrote:

"Solemnity takes possession of the mind, ... a smile of love runs over the face, ... the ebb and tide of the great ocean of reason, whose depths have never been fathomed, swell to your surging brain ... you eat and drink, and as you stand in silent amazement suns appear (where you never saw even a star) brilliant with the rays of God's wisdom, as displayed in man and the laws of life ... eternal in days ... and as true as the mind of God."

Autobiography of Andrew T. Still, page 152

THE BIODYNAMIC VIEW OF CHILDREN – PEDIATRICS THREE

Pediatrics One and Two highlight the perceptual qualities necessary to see into a child's world. We explored the Meeting Place in both. The key element is "being centered by the Health of the child." This perceptual shift, and our understanding of it, takes practice. Actually seeing the shift of our senses is the core skill—seeing that millisecond when our mind transmutes. This kind of awareness requires a content and restful mind that is capable of a precise and poised awareness. One sees details as well as the Breath of Life simultaneously. This takes some years to unfold and will only do so if the observer loves the presence of unconditional love suffusing them.

Wholeness Is Another Theme That We Have Explored.

As you know, the mind is dualistic and wants to see "pieces." Many times, Dr. Still points his listeners toward a wholeness. Embryology is slowly understanding motion as one event, not multiple fulcrums that are migrating. When we listen to a child, we try to "see" the transparency of the whole to the Breath of Life. Feel Zone B as one drop, with no distance.

Wholeness includes the Health in the child and parents as one; the family circle that the child participates in is foreign to many adults.

Endpoints in the Treatment of Children Are Acute, But the Continuum Is Long-Lasting.

Generally speaking, we overtreat and underdiagnose children. When the nature of the therapeutic force changes, then we are done ... not when all the lesions are gone or we have expansion of the Whole, as we do in adults.

Children Have an Indwelling Neutral, Very Different from That of Adults.

They almost always have retained this quality ... we call it the Desert Neutral because it is open to the "stars." So why do they need help? In fact, we all need each other, as we are one. Using outside help is normal.

In Pediatrics Three we will promote the use of decisions and direct action by the clinician ... a dangerous skill unless it is combined with a sense of the wholeness of life (Heaven). We do not retreat into our head but retain the respect and companionship of the Meeting Place. The application of force is never structural, only the use of one's attention and ease ... as you will see.

THIRD LEVEL STILLNESS AND THE MEETING PLACE

The Meeting Place is easily misinterpreted.

Our observer must be so still and neutral that the process can be seen as it happens.

Seeing the process as it happens is the key to what we are hoping to present in the idea of a Meeting Place.

This is an event that we want you to see directly, as it happens.

First, you know well that Third Level Stillness is not an end in itself ... it is a place where one waits to be healed.

Waiting here is restful ... neutral; one is not engaged in waiting.

Rest implies the sensation of being cared for, attended to as a guest ... not the host.

So one comes to the Meeting Place and becomes Neutral ... that means that one is not holding on to the stillness, but the stillness is holding the mind in a state of extreme concentration, within itself.

Many people ask me questions, and I see that some have understood holding the stillness. Holding the stillness is Level Two.

At Level Three, the stillness holds and centers you ... you feel peacefully detached from the work of being "centered in the stillness."

A neutral mind is not doing anything to promote success.

The mind is clear, undisturbed, balanced in the knowledge of creation and will. One is clear that one will be met ... but not in a predictable manner.

The host is the persona of Primary Respiration ... a living presence, not love unincarnate ... the host is the master mechanic that Dr. Still revered ... the Dad that Sutherland felt close to ...

How does the host appear?

In children, we see the presence directly, because of their transparency to the incarnate motion

of the Health ... when the love incarnating is seen ... in a millisecond we are transmuted. We are recreated ... In adults the story is a little different ... can you actually see this?

So ... one waits with no sense of responsibility at all, none ... just resting ... peacefully, relieved that one is home ... ownership of purpose and intent has ended.

Waiting becomes patience ... one can feel "I did not create myself or my fights" ... the sense of being created, not self-propelled, grows as one repeats the periods of rest and begins to love being a guest with no demands, as one realizes that the host knows even more than we do about ourselves. Then the presence of this love incarnating touches us and centers us, refines the consciousness, and the senses are converted ... we are a new and very different person from the one who sat down in Third Level Stillness ... we have been treated by the perfect physician ... and the outcome is a surprise ... we function beyond our means ... we are centered, transmuted, transparent, and empty of selfishness.

The thing I want you to see directly is ... the presence of the host and what it does to you by its presence ... can you see the process of it centering you ... not the effect, but the event of your being touched and healed so you can function in a world as yet rare to our nature. Do you see the point ... the fulcrum that moves this change ... not stillness ... but the presence of a master at your service.

It is easy to see the event this way: I was still, then I saw the Health in the child. This is not the point ... take the I's out of the sentence, so that the ego cannot fool you into a lesser reality ... there was a Third Level Stillness. I began to rest, then the rest grew ... I was not alone ...

I rested more ... not using my sense to see what was happening ... the heart became still ... there was a loving presence that overshadowed my desire to "be" ... then I was remade into a person I cherished but who was not my usual self ... another person, one transparent to the movement of love in creation of everything … after being remade and held in that state by the master's presence … I could now see the beauty and intention of his love … the mechanics of which I could not comprehend … The treatment was brief, and not something I could reproduce.

Somehow the knowledge gained did not add to the knowledge I already had, but created a love and dependency that was fearless in the face of ego and its stories … it was humbling to the point of my knowing ignorance as a meaningful place.

The point is to see the healing upon yourself as it occurs.

Why is this so hard?

One answer could be that we are not resting in Third Level Stillness … and so the story is not seen because it happens at a speed and in a place where, if we do not become neutral and rest, we will not see the main event that this teaching is trying to express.

Dr. Becker taught us, as did Still and Sutherland … "it is Deity that centers us" (1965, Dr. Becker).

We are following a legacy, and it has taken us to a great ocean where embryology, creation, and osteopathy meet … this is not easy …

It will change your life into Life.

Or … you will meet the ego, and its deceptive power will make you sure you are on track.

We are dependent on the Divine incarnate movement of love to transmute us … to recreate us as we are created to be. As this happens, we become more aware of the ego's power over us … now we begin a new phase of life … being blessed by some discernment that is two-edged … one we can feel, a loving presence, more intimate; and we can, by the same light, see our ego's role in our lives … then neutrality takes on another meaning … one of not trying to kill the enemy within but treating it the way the master does us …

Thank you …

As a practical, we can study the Third Level Stillness, The Meeting

Place, the neutral mind, the rest, the presence, the touch upon us, and the new person and sense of self that arise and are sustained by the master.

THIRD LEVEL STILLNESS IN PEDIATRICS THREE

We move deeper into First, Second, and Third Level Stillness by our response to each one. As we begin to prefer stillness to our own inner chatter and formulations, there ripens in us a discernment that unveils new kinds of stillness. Building a relationship with the Wholeness of Life requires a continuous conscious dependency that nurtures as well as creates one's ongoing existence.

As we journey into this undiscovered country we will encounter both positive and negative expressions that surprise us. We are encountering the hidden in ourselves ... in this subconscious world is both beauty and a beast ... the Health and the ego ... this is no cause for alarm, if one realizes that whatever occurs is healing and we are not the power that heals. We are neutral to what comes ... in a sense we are helpless, and we are discovering that. We are held in the hand of Love.

This unveiling gives us choices ... power or love. If we choose to let unfoldment occur, then we struggle to anchor ourselves in the proximity of a stillness we have found, until it becomes a companion. The sincerity to be Neutral ripens.

As we repattern our senses, a new stillness appears, and the old stillness seems less potent.

This walk along the pathway home is one of the absolutes becoming relative ... the magnitude of the potency of the stillness increases until it becomes fierce in its transmutation of our being.

Third Level Stillness is so powerful and potent that it immediately (in seconds) changes who and what one is. It centers us, converts our senses and holds them on center. The display before us is a relief, as weariness and a false sense of responsibility perish, so fast that no memory is retained … all one knows is the sense of being made, now, along with everything.

The amazing conversion of the senses has mercifully occurred through the power of the Third Level Stillness … now the whole idea of effort is inverted into a true dependency … this then creates a new personal history, and a new story appears … one that has always been present … only hidden from our awareness. Now choice is not desired. One is known as beloved by the Beloved; again the distance narrows …

Third Level Stillness is a landscape. To traverse it, we must commit to the task of crossing "undiscovered country" … unremembered trails and scenery … we travel naked, transparent to the sea around us … The sensation of the "House Under the Sea" slowly becomes our sense of being … the soma begins to reform, juxtaposed to the spirit of the house and distancing itself from the chaos of the "House of Babel" … crossing the great plains of this new landscape changes how one "works" …

One anchors oneself to the silent sea without being persuaded or distracted by either good intentions or fears. One clings to it as a domain.

At first, one must use discipline and concentration to remain here. The past and the future end at this doorway.

The room behind one's breathing becomes a room as big as the sea. The breathing is not in them, but through everything … the mode of prayer and meditation shifts to the outside presence of life and the interior presence of a shelter for birth. One *remembers* more than one *does.*

This Third Level Stillness, if cherished as reality, will ripen and unveil the truth in our relationships with children.

When we are met by this beauty, the potency of the flow into us makes a big change in our interior world and being. Our senses hook up to Health, and we see, hear, smell, touch, and taste a new world that is also sensing us. This reversal of the senses is called a spiritual conversion of the more temporal sensorium into one that is oriented to the Health and Eternity.

We are mingled with the flow of creation ... here in this place of creation, one sometimes sees the angels, or feels like one is in a glass globe filled with silence that is unaltered by the movements of time or civilization ...

One enters a waiting room filled with Third Level Stillness ... one waits ... one becomes neutral, active without doing ... a child gazes toward you ... the gaze is seen, a meeting occurs. The meeting causes love to show itself ... the silence crescendos into angelic proportions (Fourth Level Stillness) ... outside, the movement of the storm is tossing everything about (the lesion, distractions), but the space of eternity is untouched by the passing of these events ... one is sheltered from the storm. The storm is human nature ... yours as well as others.

The event is Wholeness and Eternity woven into incarnation.

There are a variety of events that cause the conversion of the senses ... sometimes a sound from a child, a smile, the joy of their freedom; sometimes they look through us and introduce us to our Health.

The task that we are pointing toward here is to see the moment of conversion ... we want to see it happen, see ourselves carried across the bridge ... it is not enough to see the effect, the outcome ... can you see the transmutation of your perception as it occurs?

This will make all the difference in how you make this state of being more of who you are ... it builds a specific kind of humility and memory that eliminates the sense that you "have a skill" that is at all independent of the Divine Tide of innocence, love, and its gift to you of life ... all of it.

Thank you.

Recommended reading

"Be Still and Know." This is a dedication to William G. Sutherland, D.O., presented in Philadelphia, Pennsylvania, on September 22, 1965, by Rollin Becker, D.O.

Here are the first few lines. Find the whole presentation and read it slowly. It is included in *Life in Motion: The Osteopathic Vision of Rollin E. Becker, D.O.* What is Dr. Becker pointing to?

> The theme of this paper is the continuous recognition of the necessity of "being still in order to know" through the most direct Channel possible, that of being closer to your Maker than mere material breathing. It should also have as a supplement to the title, "Be Still and Know, a re-dedication to William G. Sutherland." When one thinks of a dedication to a man who has given a great service to mankind, there is a tendency to think of it as something that happened when he was alive and that this is a new day, and filled with new discoveries. A re-dedication, on the other hand, is a living thing, a continuing experience, an unfolding understanding, and the promise of greater truths to follow. …

A STILL SMALL VOICE

Dr. Becker referred to these words many times. He insisted upon not adding to what the Tide transmitted. He asked us to "be still and know that I am God" (Psalm 46:10, KJV).

Dr. Becker was transmitting deep truths from the ancient wisdom of prophets. Psalm 46 is from King David when he is struck mute by the hand of God. God speaks to him and stills him. It is important to know that the "being still" in this case was not an act of human will. It was a highly elevated state of recognition of an individual by God, bringing that person into union and enlightenment. It is the most sacred state of being, in all traditions.

Around 800 BC, Elijah, a poor desert dweller, enters the flock of the Judeo-Christian tradition. He obviously was impoverished by choice, like the desert dwellers that followed him years later. He was dressed for survival. He was not a priest. He was homeless, poor, and unkempt.

The belief of the Jews at that time was that God would speak only to the religious leaders. There was a firm hierarchy that one had to recognize in order to be in the presence of God. There was a belief in the "chosen few." Elijah confronted these inequalities.

He told the masses that God was within them. That God spoke in a still small voice inside the heart of everyone.

In Elijah's time this was something new for most people, something that was contrary to thousands of years of tradition. Elijah awakens us to an indwelling place of God's presence ... and a direct communication therein ... what we call conscience.[1]

---

[1] The word "conscience" means to know together with God as one. Why would Dr. Becker point us here to these ancient teachers?

Is this not the Health, which we have pursued in our tradition?

There are no chosen few ... there is a voice ... a still and small voice ... how can we understand the wordless voice ... why is it so small, like an embryo? All these questions are answerable inside your own temple (Health).

The greatest step is being centered by deity ... letting yourself be healed, reconstructed by love.

God is Love.

THE MEMORY OF ETERNITY

The soma has a strong orientation toward normal.

We generally, in the Western culture, divide ourselves into body, soul, and spirit. The body, when intimate with the Health, is transparent and is called soma. This word is from ancient Sanskrit ... In my understanding, the word conveys an image of a tree growing beside the river of life.

As we begin to feel the Health and have a sensory experience of it, the body begins to crave stillness and the embrace of the presence that the Health transmits. This is like a beacon for the body, calling it to a rich and whole sensory life. The body becomes enamored with the beloved Health. It wants to get back home.

As the body forms a memory of the sensations of the Health, it naturally moves toward the spirit of the Health ... the Imago Dei. There is a constant movement toward the perfect midline.

This memory of eternity is always there but is often overshadowed by the more temporal memory of the brain synapses formed genetically and culturally.

The soul is an ambivalent duality. It is the seat of the ego and self-centered desires. When the body moves toward the spirit, the ego fights to keep its dominion over the body. The brain-mind then appears to be more agitated, because it is. The domination of years is now challenged, not directly, but the ego does not want to lose its kingdom.

As you work with children, you must remember that what they "are" is also in you... here are some hints that helped me:

Do not resist the ego, except with more stillness and dependency on the Divine.

When you place your hands on a child, ask your hands to remember the sensation of the Health, the sensation of eternity. The hands want to go there ... the psyche will not be very helpful, as it fears the dissolution of its existence.

Let your hands be embryonic ... use the beauty of the embryo to remind the hands.

Doctor the voltage until you feel the beauty. Voltage in your hands comes from willpower.

Remember that we are transparent to the movement of the Breath of Life, which is Love.

A NORMAL CHILD

They have no structure, only form, dying and becoming.

Children are a living dynamic, not a static structure. We are not like trees, which place layer upon layer. This ever-changing form is not the addition of substance to an anatomical infrastructure that expands ... the changes occur as the old forms die, and the new form is printed in the Fluid Body.

The image and pattern of unfoldment appear at conception. Life is the unfoldment of the blueprint ... if ... the Fluid Body is healthy and vital. This means, among other things, that it can rebalance and establish neutral as it swings from the old into the new. The change is powered by the potency (fire) of Primary and Thoracic Respiration (fire). Through this, one meets milestones that express the moving dynamic.

Think about the difference between a train passing as you watch ... and one that is sitting still on the tracks.

Children form two million synapses per minute during their early years ... two million. This kind of speed is going on under our hands, with such precision and wholeness that, unless we change our observational bias, we will miss the osteopathy at work.

Children are never the same for two days in a row ... watch and you will see the drama of unfoldment ... they change and they adapt to constant "newness" ... making adults look like stalled engines.

These processes go on throughout life. Think about how you grow as an adult ... it depends on your capacity for Neutral.

The First Breath

This commentary is about osteopathic vital signs related to the first breath and how that breath creates momentum for present and future health issues.

Little is written on this subject, but the oral teaching has been passed on for decades. All the basic courses I've attended (twelve) mentioned the first breath.

The person who made the most sense to me was Dr. Fulford. He focused on the long-term sequelae in children who had not completed the first breath—those who were desynchronized for the unity of all breaths being one when we enter this world.

From his direction and insight, I pursued this topic in many ways for many years ... I have used it for thirty years ... it is very practical knowledge, in spite of the spiritual overtones.

The first earthly breath of a newborn is always a moment of marvelous beauty and relief.

The wholeness of the movement of the breaths through the birthing as a whole creates an individual aligned consciously with the Health and able to function freely. These words coming from Dr. Fulford were few and valued.

What did he mean?

My understanding, while talking to him, was based upon my knowledge of the mystical path he had followed and what the words "whole," "individual," "consciously aligned," and "free-willed" would mean in the inner world ...

Children are remarkably complete, whole, and free. They unfold from the blueprint of life set at conception. In order for development to unfold continuously, one must have a well-established fulcrum between Primary Respiration, thoracic respiration, and ignition.

At the time of the first breath after birth, the demands of life increase severely ... the ignition creates more fire, the Tide orchestrates, the Dynamic Stillness pours in through the midline, and as the air rushes into the lungs, one breath is set in time as eternity comes ashore. The feeling is wholeness, not parts. If one feels parts, then there is a lesion.

To be an individual, in Dr. Fulford's terminology, means to follow the destiny of unfoldment, not worldly images. The journey for Dr. Fulford was to listen to the love behind creation and follow its voice. The result of this hard work would be that one becomes what God made them for, not what one's genetics and ego might overlay.

The first breath establishes memory and the vital oneness that carries one's name. If the first breath is weak, our struggle to know ourselves may be extended and spiritual maturity delayed (prolonging the sense of isolation from life).

To be consciously aligned means, in the context of his work, to be aware of Divine will and to have an instinctual need to be in the presence of love and perfection. This is the Self of the immune system.

Free will, as Dr. Fulford put it, is when one has no slavery to habits or beliefs. One is free to be shifted by the movement of the Creator's hand. One is free to lighten the load of world suffering. One is detached, impartial to everything, neutral and responsive to the unfoldment of God's love. This is not a willy-nilly going with the flow ... it is love meeting love with no preconceived outcome. It is fearless in the face of one's timidity.

In the biodynamic view, the first breath is relative, not absolute.

The first true breath is at or before conception. Obviously Thoracic Respiration (O_2 metabolic exchange) begins much earlier than birth.

The presence of Primary Respiration guiding conception is a biodynamic principle that emerges from both osteopathy and embryology.

The birthing breath is the first earthly breath and, ideally, thoracic, primary, and the ignition move together as one.

Think about the capacity of Zone B to do its work, to accomplish unfoldment of the blueprint of life, if the first breath is desynchronized and weakened. Can it follow the outpouring of the movement of life as it grows, if it has no power to do so?

The first hint of this, if you are not trained to see it through Fluid Body dynamics, is slowness in the remolding of the head after birth. This should be a red flag that there is a problem in the core. Not plagiocephaly … but a delay in the rapid remolding of the head after birth … At seventy-two hours the head should be remolded. For many, twenty-four hours is sufficient.

At conception, the Divine image is breathed into protoplasm (clay). The perfect image is made, and we call it the Health. This is a lifelong reference point for normal that is indispensable for healing and unfoldment. Without this, life does not move forward. It stagnates.

Protoplasm is the first moldable substance that can hold an image (Oxford English Dictionary) and the image is unerring in its timing and geometry. The inscription is immortal. This is, for me, the first breath … some mothers feel it as they conceive.

This could be called the absolute first breath.

Reflection on this surpasses the written history of human life.

Each of us must think about these truths in light of the clinical and personal outcomes we experience day to day in our work.

In pediatrics, we will return to this topic, as it is very important to know what normal is for a child, because Primary Respiration is so different in adults.

BIRTH

Fire

Ignition

Thoracic Respiration

Divine Breath

One Breath

Incarnation Unfolds

One Is Borne.

ONE BREATH

Practical

Evaluate the connection between the Movement of Eternity, Thoracic Respiration, and Primary Respiration in an adult.

Is there one breath?

If not, rebalance by going to the Health and waiting in the light.

THE FLAME OF INTENTION

One of Dr. Sutherland's goals was to communicate with the Tide. As you know, he labored long and hard to free himself from the "physical senses," as he called them. As he did, new horizons opened. He began to recognize the Tide as an effect of a supreme and loving intelligence. He then realized that the will and intention of God could be realized.

This awakening did not occur overnight; it was the effect of a great effort to think independently of what he knew. It was also the outcome of faith in the Tide and being neutral enough to let it center him.

"Thinking osteopathy" leads us into new landscapes. As we enter these places, we are healed by the presence of the Tide. This healing changes our sense from a materialistic reductionist convergent function into a sense reconnected to the Health, and we see life in a very different way. As this change occurs, we begin at times to see that the world is transparent to the Breath of Life ... that everything is moving from one eternal source. Love and creation eternally in motion. This realization is a beautiful shock, one that changes our thinking and our sense of normality.

These changes are not automatic; one must wish for less internal chaos and want to be healed. This requires a practical faith in the Tide, a trust that allows change, change that is not predictable. The ego, in its laziness, will resist, and so it takes many years to find oneself empty of willfulness and filled with a soft joy, silence, peace, and neutrality.

A relationship with the mover of the Tide helps many patients, who would otherwise benefit much less from any other method available in medicine today. It also allows entry into the world of children that is clinically miles ahead of the more rigid formats.

The "flame of intention" is a therapeutic force that can be seen in every patient (as the Tide permits). It can communicate to us the intention of the Breath of Life. It also reveals a precise look at its laser-like "noninvasive surgical skill" at a cellular level. The flame will communicate its intention clearly and will demonstrate that intention without you adding any intention of your own other than attentiveness to the flame.

The intention is not a conclusion from what you see, but a transmission from the wisdom of the flame.

THE FLAME

Practical

Notice that everything is transparent to the Breath of Life. There is a wind passing through everything. It is the motion of creation, the eternal motion of Divine love.

If this is not easily noticed, look outside in nature for a while, then at the patient, with divergent vision, vision that does not focus anywhere. If this does not help, sit in Third Level Stillness for a while, and let it help you to a neutrality of the senses.

Trust your judgment. If it is a fantasy, then the treatment will not work. Take the risk to trust what you see and embrace it.

Go to the patient and place your hands on the flame. Make sensory contact and mold your hands to the shape, with the longest finger abutting the tip of the flame.

Physically follow the flame and listen to it ... focus your attention with great care.

It will demonstrate a treatment at many levels.

It will stop without making the patient perfect.

The flame does not go out but recedes into a liquid light.

The treatment continues for many days. Try to predict how long.

Let the patient rest.

Wholeness is a word with no meaning.

Wholeness is beauty radiant with Divine presence. Wholeness only exists in an ocean of eternity that carries any sense of self into the I Am of God spoken in everything at once. The experience overshadows any attempt at definition. It is known by its presence and by its effect on the witness.

How does this fit into osteopathy?

Osteopathy is grounded in the realization of a Supreme Intelligence creating all of life.

The embryology that I studied earlier in my life has changed into a field of science that is proving, to the rational mind, the truth of Dr. Still's principles of osteopathy. Earlier in my life I studied embryonic segmentation, which gives rise to the integrative function of the autonomic nervous system as a whole. Unlesioned autonomic function is invisible. Invisible but beautiful, often giving the observer a sense of tremendous peace and harmony, peace and harmony that is not "in" the patient but through everything.

Awareness of normal is a deeply spiritual moment when one's observer is burned away by love. As we study the sensation of normal, we arrive at a point where palpitation ends and sensing reaches deep into the reality behind the processing of the parts. We come to an awareness of a homogenized whole, transparent to cause. Our study of the dysfunction of the autonomic nervous system has allowed us to bring it to balance, and in doing so, exposed us to wholeness rarely seen with any scientific tool, other than our indwelling sense. Still said that our "skill is proportionate to our understanding of normal." What we have come to see is how true this is. Our goal in treatment cannot reach beyond what we consider "normal" for the end point. Over the years, I have clearly seen the limits that I have placed on normal by my reductionist frameworks and fears of reaching beyond my limits. Since I let the Tide center me, all the fear has been replaced by love and dependency. Normal is a Mystery. A great thing of beauty, not some state in the parts. It is Wholeness, the meaning of which transcends knowing.

The great osteopaths (those with exceptional clinical outcomes using only their hands) all point us toward this beauty, this Wholeness. Generally our professional groups are afraid and shun these realities. I have heard many voices that feel pain when these ideas are expressed. Many are angry at any idea that does not fit in their understanding ... this attitude is classified as neurotic and should be avoided by all of us. It has and is destroying the profession.

My personal despair with these voices was relieved by Bill Johnston, D.O., who contributed much to osteopathy. He was a pioneer in communication with ease, wholeness, neutral, and indirect action. He did not like the direct approach of Magoun. He was inspired to find more healing with less mental and manual force. After I gave a lecture on the death of osteopathy, he was very upset with me ... he believed I was damning the profession. I called him and explained that the goal of the lecture was about accepting the death, not causing it. Our discussion was successful and we became very open and truthful with each other. I asked him to describe for me the end point of the perfect functional method of treatment. He was silent ... out of his silence rose a stillness. The pause between us was long. After a few minutes he spoke: "You would not believe it," he said. I did not respond, as the Tide was still filling me. Finally I said, "Thank you, Bill." The click of the phone faded in the air of love. He was a teacher, one that could take you into experience. In this case, we went to a place of Wholeness, the end point where healing enters the realms of what Still did and proposed to us. Bill showed me what we all have in common as osteopaths. Where we all merge from our separate doorways and biases ... he and I journeyed into common ground and beyond the entry point of our friction.

Wholeness is not a word with any meaning.

The meaning comes from the witnessing of wholeness after a long and personal healing from living with the tides of life. Bill Johnston communicated wholeness directly. Functional methodology and biodynamic methodology both seek to bring wholeness to the surface and transmute the veil that our lesions have created in ourselves and others.

Can we say that the hopeful end point of treatment is wholeness?

Yes ... because the end point is beautiful and serene, and ... no ... because lesions are part of the wholeness that is present, whether we perceive it or not ... therein is the reason wisdom cannot be captured by logic or definition, where there is a great mystery in life, and the more you know, the more you know the limits of being human.

Wholeness is not in individual parts, people, or pieces ... it is one reality behind the veil of several.

A CHILD'S SENSE OF WHOLENESS

Children's experience of wholeness is alive. For adults the memory of this is limp.

Children feel a family circle and are intent on being in it ... often they bring the adults into it, and a new Zone B is felt by the adults, which transcends the individual Zone B. We will discuss this as a topic and as a practice.

Children are very much aware of things that many adults search for.

When you treat, hold the child's sense of wholeness in your heart ... let it lead you on to your own recollection and the spatial dynamics of the child's awareness.

Children also know the oneness of the spiritual family formed by all children ... they even have a universal language.

When we treat a particular child and are aware of all the children who will never be treated ... who have no access to help ... then we open a doorway to seeing into their world ... a little. There is plenty of love in the "mechanism" for everyone ... do not crowd the awareness of a child ... they can lead you without dismissing your help and treatment.

Again, we will do a practical with this intention ... at some point.

You Should Treat Adults as Children.

A MOMENT OF GREAT CHANGE

As many people know, I worked with Ruby Day, D.O., every two weeks at her home near where I lived for many, many years.

She was with Sutherland from 1938 until his passing. She taught with him and was a member of his private study group. After he died, she refused to follow Magoun and stayed on the periphery. She was a country doctor in a small town, where she was loved as an icon of service.

Ruby was petite and present, always prepared with a lesson plan. She guided me past many falsities in myself and my thinking as an osteopath.

After ten years with her, at the end of a teaching session for me, she said, "I would like you to treat me," in a questioning tone of voice…

I was a little taken aback but joyfully consented.

We went to her bedroom, and she lay supine. I cradled her head in what was known as the "Becker hold"… she came to neutral.

As she did, she said, "Now, treat me as if I was newborn."

As she drifted deeper into the Tide, I was given the awareness to feel her as if she was a newborn.

Her head was made of soft transparent fluid as rich in content as that of a new child… I trusted her… she was unparalleled as a teacher. What I saw, I believed immediately… yes, the Health is always there.

Here was an eighty-year-old woman whose therapeutics were exactly like a newborn's… I had been taught in courses how different children were from adults.

Now, in one moment, my whole thinking and being was shifted to seeing that adults could be treated as one would treat a child…

When I left, she was sleeping… I think.

IMAGES OF THE HEALTH FROM STILL AND SUTHERLAND

Children are transparent to the Health.

These words are paramount to the treatment of children in the Biodynamic Method.

Certainly Dr. Still posed a very profound truth when he said, "Find the Health; anyone can find disease." ... What does this mean? ... What is it like to experience the Health in oneself and others? ... Has anyone described it?

Drs. Still and Sutherland both describe an experience of the Health.

At eighty-six years of age, Dr. Still said, "I love my patients. I see God in their faces and their form."

These words are not timid. Dr. Still was straightforward. He was not looking at lesions. How did he come to this "ability"? I do not know.

I can report on how this has happened for thousands of osteopaths and myself, practitioners who do see the Health, the Divine, and a movement of life in their patients.

My introduction was from Dr. Becker personally and in his 1965 Sutherland Memorial Lecture about the spiritual fulcrum. He states, "The Deity centers us." This refers to the Divine centering us ... it's not that we center ourselves. This awareness is common in contemplative practices that appreciate our inner poverty; "it is by the grace of God that we can perceive the invisible work of the Spirit." There is a distinct awareness when this happens to us. We are transformed in seconds from our own content to being an effect of another, deeply loving presence. Our effort must have ceased in order for us to see the moment of impregnation and a total change in being.

Still was clear that human intelligence has severe limits without the intercession of a higher mind.

To witness the Health in another person, one's senses must be transmuted by the Health itself touching one's being when one is neutral. This was made clear to me by Rollin Becker when he looked at me one day and said, "Do not begin your treatment until the will of the patient surrenders to the will of Primary Respiration!" He was very direct and concrete as he said this. I was shocked. He had taken the end point of treatment, as I understood it, and made it the beginning. After many years, his guidance became clear and profound.

The treatment begins when there is a sustained neutral in the whole. Children have this most of the time. Even sick children are transparent to the Health. This transparency is a special kind of neutral that is persistent in children in spite of their disease. Children do not lose their capacity to love, even when they are critically ill. Adults, as you know, change their moods with their sense of wellness. You will find that even very ill children will center you. They transmit the flow of the Divine.

When we are in a neutral that is saturated with Third Level Stillness, we become receptive in a unique manner. We are neutral, waiting serenely for the Tide to enter the moment and unveil to the senses the invisible world of the Health. This is the "deity centering us," creating a new level of awareness ... In working with children, because they are deeply suffused by the Divine and the incarnate Health, their mere presence is enough to center us and bring our senses to "seeing" the Health ... if ... we are neutral and at the "Meeting Place," i.e., Third Level Stillness.

This requires a certain inner awareness of the many ways we can fool ourselves.

As we are, our senses operate from the self-centered mind of our self-image. What does this mean? The synapses in our brain develop around familial and cultural interchanges. As children and young adults, we have many projections placed on us. From these trillions of synapses, we form a synthetic center ... one we create from the world around us, not the one in us from the beginning of life.

Many of us are working to "find our Health and discover ourselves" as we were originally made. That is to say, "to see God's face and form in ourselves and others," as Dr. Still stated.

Our senses, as we are, are attached to the ego, and so we see others as projections of our own classifications, not as transparent beings reflecting the Divine image of the Health. We are all doing this. This understanding helps us to comprehend neutrality and to make a choice to allow "Deity to center us" ...

Children will do this for us ... if we meet them at the Meeting Place. The transparency of children is that they are "empty" and transparent to the movement of creation. We see a transcendent love entering through them, creating/healing the cellular unfoldment of the child.

This appreciation of a simple and clear awareness of creation is part of the legacy we receive from Drs. Still and Sutherland. Let's review their teachings.

Dr. Still refers to mind/motion/matter.

Dr. Still said that these laws are not "framed by human hands."

The mind he speaks of is the Supreme Intelligence of the Divine Mystery. This Mystery animates as the Breath of Life (i.e., motion), which incarnates as the material world (matter). Thus we have Spirit moving into creation and unfolding the blueprint of life. We can see this if we are "centered by the Tide." When centered, we can see mind, motion, and creation as a singularity of the movement of life as a whole.

The sensation of eternity entering time is beauty. Sutherland and others follow the lead of Still.

In the first edition of Magoun's *Osteopathy in the Cranial Field,* Sutherland reports both his view and Still's view of the Health, a transparent wholeness without systems or parts. Remember, this is not philosophy, but the report of direct perceptual activity.

"Motion must be guided by a supreme being down to the individual cell, otherwise there would be chaos and death" (A. T. Still).

Sutherland then quotes Still again:

"Dr. Still understood the cerebral spinal fluid as the highest known element in the human body. He envisioned this fluid as an intermediary in the movement of Divine intelligence ... a channeling of creation into embryological segments and irrigating them with life ... giving form and function, order and intelligence, to our existence. All life is manifest in this motion" (see page 15, paragraphs 1 and 2).

This is what we see when we awaken to the Health ...

In *Contributions of Thought,* Sutherland again addresses a simple picture of Wholeness (see April 12, 1948):

Here Sutherland describes feeling the CSF and the Breath of Life (the movement of Supreme Intelligence) ... feeling the spark of life that ignites the potency. An unerring, overshadowing, and superseding function that he called Primary Respiration.

He sees a dynamic interchange (as mentioned by Dr. Becker) between creation and the created ... These impressions came to Sutherland only after he stopped using force!

Later in life, Dr. Sutherland asked his wife to paint a picture of Primary Respiration as he experienced it. Again, another image appears that mimics those we have just discussed:

A "House Under the Sea".

The painting was lost in political bickering, but the story has been told to me by three of my mentors, Ruby Day, Anne Wales, and John Harakal. Recently, I was told by a historian that the house in the painting was A. T. Still's cabin ... that would suggest a very deep love and remembrance of his teacher.

The "House Under the Sea" is biodynamic, in the sense that this image is similar to Blechschmidt's insistence that we are formed from a mysterious force coming through us from the "outside." The similarity with Still, Sutherland, and the foundation of osteopathy in embryology is what prompted me to choose the name "Biodynamics of Osteopathy." The commonality of images provoked by all these observant men is heartwarming to anyone who has felt these things and feels a little crazy when told that there is only structure in osteopathic diagnosis and treatment.

The image of a house transparent to the ocean of the Breath of Life brings again the sensory experience of transparency, of something passing through us, unimpeded, that heals/creates as it passes without diminishing itself. This Supreme Intelligence is the Master Mechanic, the Physician Within, the Health, the Higher Self, and the Divine Image in all of Life.

Children are the archetype of normality, radiant with these truths.

Our elders saw these truths ... we can approach their teaching only when we are neutral and free to be centered by Deity ... this is why we call it the "Meeting Place."

EVALUATION OF THE CENTRAL NERVOUS SYSTEM

A Biodynamic Summary

In a Healthy child, no parts are discernible.

Each separate activity is evaluated for internal disengagement under the influence of the Tide.

Synchronization with the Tide
(Check for paradoxical motion)
Augmentation with other motions of the system
(Check for contradictory motions)
Transmutation of the function toward Neutral

Activities to evaluate:

The sacs ... (periosteal, dural, brain proper) and the neural tube
Bowing of the tadpole into the "sea around us"
The tadpole as a whole moving toward lamina terminalis during inhalation (only with rates)
Coiling in the lateral ventricles toward lamina terminalis during the inhalation period
Rocking on the waterbeds
The bird
Ignition
Motion present of reciprocal tension potency in ventricle 3
CNS fluid field
CNS collective reciprocal tension potency

Sacral rise with the inhalation period; this includes tissue, fluid, and reciprocal tension potency

The effect of Thoracic Respiration on the brain and fluid cisterns

There is a Whole that will appear when the Tide deems it. It is not a vision of all the parts but a transparency that is unlimited and capable of communication.

HOLY CHILDREN

Being with Children

The world is full of advice about children. This commentary is not advice.

Children are incarnating into time and circumstances, and we as adults may fail to see this in the light of what it means to the Wholeness of life.

Children, If They Are Lucky, Grow.

Each milestone a child reaches brings a sigh of relief from anyone who has been in a children's clinic and has seen the suffering that befalls many innocents.

Our Job Is to Be at the Door Before a Lesion Appears as a Disease.

When a child walks, it is the effect of a precision of unfolding that is profound and unerring in its form and function (timing).

The science of growth and development called embryology contains a great mystery that will astound you. Understanding and engaging this mystery will also perhaps remove any sense that your child needs your guidance to crawl or walk or develop any physiological function. It is indwelling.

Let me say that the unfolding of the pattern of growth is unstoppable unless there is a stress on the process from a distinct source—a source which may or may not be identifiable.

As a devoted contemplative and one who praises Socratic ignorance, I have watched children from my professional perch for nearly 40 years.

What I've seen would fill volumes.

What I have concluded is that we as adults need to be trained to be with children on their terms ... to find their place of reference, not ours.

I was with a ten-month-old child in a store ... the child became restless. I could feel that he was overloaded ... we went outside and sat on a bench at the intersection of the city center, a noisy, chaotic place. We sat ... together. A stillness descended from above onto us ... it came from afar ... we were held in it for fifteen minutes, being instantaneously filled to the brim with love.

Neither of us moved; the grace held us.

Beside us on the bench was a man reading a newspaper, unhappy with the unchanging nature of the news. Around us were people, people all moving in individual directions ... no one saw the fiery cocoon. We were not distracted by all that was happening around us.

The child was still, and totally relaxed without moving during the whole fifteen minutes ... when the beauty passed, he moved gently but did not seem to have lost a sense of presence as I had.

He had led me to the moment, but I had to be available, and that is the core issue we need to address in ourselves as adults, practitioners, or family members.

We need to be present to the child on their terms and have a wish to try to be responsive from that viewpoint rather than our own role ideologies.

Ask a mother what she hears from the child during birth.

Can anyone see self-healing forces at work as a child plays or sleeps?

Does a child schedule meditation?

I am with an eleven-month-old. He is very forceful and playing hard. Without any sensible clue that I can note, he suddenly shifts from intense physical play to resting his head on my thigh and looking out the window ... in a millisecond he shifted his affect from play to an intensely soft concentration of looking into Eternity as if the world was transparent to his gaze through it into Heaven.

He was seeing through the temporal.

I could feel him incarnating as the Fluid Body swirled out the design of a new form. He was not only feeling this movement but also the source, which I could not feel.

All I noted was a stillness of Holy content and the physical sense of eternity. I was returning toward my death as he was unfolding into life, our paths crossing ... him coming ... me going ... on the same fulcrum.

As osteopaths with a motive to find the indwelling self-healing forces, we have come to recognize Primary Respiration, and have pursued it and it us ... we are just beginning to see the laws of healing in a new way.

It requires that we be neutral with the readiness to be shifted by the great Tide at any second ... a dependency of being that denies ownership of self or others and enjoys ignorance.

Someone was overheard explaining to another parent how she had taught her child to walk ... this was her glory ... what she had done for the child ... I pray that not too many of us take credit for what is given. This is a place of great loss in the way we see events ... let's watch ourselves and see if we steal the credit for what we do not do, but is done, not through us, but in everything.

Two children, pre-walkers, pass each other in their strollers ... the adults pushing ... the children gaze at each other, longingly silent ... transfixed.

They have never seen each other before ... they commune, perhaps speak some forgotten language ... we perhaps notice this ... numb to the content ... are they talking?

Do they recognize their beingness as one?

What questions could we ask? They are adult questions, about something we cannot access with a question ... we are ignorant, a step into wisdom and beauty.

Do we have an essential language we all know, when we stop everything that is familiar and controllable?

Does it have sound?

I wonder.

The journey into the unknown with a child is not a passing experience, a pleasant memory ... it is a relationship with Life, the death and birth of each moment ... this is how a child becomes and grows, if left to the given resources that we are all endowed with ...

We take this journey if we wish to be free of the chains of assumption.

A child, twelve months old, reaches toward a cat, the hand in slow motion like it was moving underwater ... the fingers motionless ... As the hand comes to a single whisker ... the cat remains motionless ... A finger unfolds from the child's hand like a spring fern ... slowly the touch comes; no one moves. Beauty suffuses the moment.

Why so slow?

Again, another adult question ... there are no answers. First we must live in the child's world, and for adults that may take some training.

We begin with Third Level Stillness, a dynamic where the eternal enters time. Here we can sense the child and the effects upon it ... when we listen for the call from the mantle of this stillness, we can begin to taste a Meeting Place.

Fourteen months

Closing the latch of a child's car seat, I say, "I will love you forever," into the preciousness ... he kisses me ... I go around into the driver's seat ... I sit ... as I come to rest in the seat ... a crescendo of fire into the heart

… the smallness of the wave was from its purity and lack of materiality … sweet beyond any sensation this world has to offer … a wisp of a whisper.

ONENESS

Practical

Sit in groups of three … go to Third Level Stillness and be neutral and ready … still, but vital … but neutral to outcomes … ready for the Tide of transmutation.

Wait until you disappear and oneness comes into the group. Oneness does not come from participation or clarity.

The Tide is there, already creating. What you see as good or bad effort is useless … be neutral.

Thank you.

THREE LEVELS OF STILLNESS

Practical

Sit in small groups of three or four ... with persons you do not know very well.

As individuals ... slowly explore in yourself the three levels of stillness. Notice how you approach the solution. Try to find each one.

Be neutral ... patiently indifferent.

Watch.

Wait.

What transpires?

THE "LOCKED-UP" HEAD

Not infrequently we see children with "locked-up" heads. This means that everything is compressed and not moving. The head and all layers of function are like cement.

Certainly we want to make sure the Fluid Body is functioning. In these cases the compression in the head is overwhelming.

There is something I do that I find very useful and rewarding.

From the pelvis (the sacrum in adults) move the fluid, tissue, bones, and reciprocal tension potency gently toward lamina terminalis, when the Tide tells you. Move everything as one, and make sure that the tissues, fluid, and "fluid in the fluid" move as one, not separately.

You will feel a response in the head. One of the inner functions or layers will release a little. This motion can now be engaged as motion present or as a doorway through which the Tide will guide you.

This is called "putting slack in the system."

The practical in adults is done through the sacral area using no force and engaging perception through Third Level Stillness.

NO RESPONSE TO TREATMENT

"Your skill is proportionate to your understanding of normal" – Dr. Still

This aphorism by our teacher is something to meditate upon. Take a second or two and think ... is my skill focused on an awareness of normal function, or am I perhaps identifying with lesion removal or tenacity? Let's stop and feel intuitively, what is my skill interfacing with in my mind? ... what is the message I am sending to my hands? What is the motive driving my relationship with the child? Watch yourself and see who is in control.

A lack of response to treatment can be frustrating ... remember, this is where we really learn from the mechanism, from the teacher ... If we are seeking to learn more and more concerning the indwelling work of Primary Respiration, then failure of the patient to respond to the treatment means we must watch and learn how the mechanism is trying to accomplish resolution.

Watch.

Do not probe for solutions.

Listen ... what are the healing forces working toward?

How?

Watch ... what is missing in the lesion ... what aspect of normal is not present?

Wait ... watch ... Ruby Day and others have told me that Dr. Sutherland watched sometimes for 45 minutes ... what was he doing? ... Dr. Rollin Becker would speak to us about waiting, watching, until that "still small voice spoke."

Assess your perceptual habits ... this is the first step in difficult cases.

Did you rush in "where angels fear to tread"?

No response requires another fresh look at the levels of Fluid Body activity.

Is there something you did not consider?

Review the history ... again and again ... chemicals, immunizations, alcohol, nicotine, medications, do you suspect abuse? ... Listen in the pauses between the words of the answers you receive; where does that lead you?

A child that had severe eczema and Fluid Body dysfunction but felt healthy, failed to respond to treatment (one) ... I knew I had missed something obvious, but I obviously did not know what ... I went back over the history again and again ... until finally, I found out the child was sleeping on vinyl ... and that there was no ventilation in the room ... We attended to this, and she was promptly well. I did not treat her a second time until I had reviewed every aspect of her day. Open windows are necessary for everyone. Cheap vinyl gives off toxic gas.

A "floppy fluid" can happen when there is no organization of the reciprocal tension potency into a form that gives the fluid integrity ... here one must ask, "What is missing?" "Floppy fluid" feels lifeless and too "loose" ... it has no power. The ignition is on hot. Somehow the receptivity of the fluid is blocked. The only thing I could think of when I first saw this was to do a CV4 ... Sutherland used this procedure to reorganize the "fluid in the fluid," i.e., reciprocal tension potency. When I tried this as a last attempt to help the situation, nothing transpired. Nothing! Then I listened more than thinking ... listened to how the system was trying to act rather than discover "how do I fix it" ... then ... there was a clear sense of the Fluid Body trying, however unsuccessfully, to do a CV4/EV4 in the whole body at the same time!

I did manage to do both at once, and the results were helpful. What does it mean to have no integrity and to need both CV4 and EV4 at once? What I think is that, because children have no rates and because CV4 and EV4 are the same process, any direction given to "in or out" is in a sense giving a rate to the Fluid Body. There is a demand for all directions at once.

In another type of case there is the opposite: "a locked-up system." Inertia reigns! No motion anywhere.

Here we have situations where we cannot motion test (not that we need to) without creating acute symptoms (i.e., seizure activity, etc.). In these rare cases, one can put "slack into the system" as a whole, to find motion present.

A LETTER ABOUT COMMUNICATION AND CHILDREN

Dear Dr. Jealous,

When my girlfriend found out she was pregnant she had a dream that I was treating her, and communicating with the baby.

She booked in and told me ... I thought it was strange; I usually do not communicate with babies separate from the mom.

The first treatment at ten weeks was about moving through the fear, a lot of it, some mine, some hers, some from her social surroundings.

The second treatment she was much calmer. It was a very deep and still treatment. The baby thanked me for looking after his mom.

Then he taught me what his hands feel like as an embryo. He showed me I still have these hands myself. How can it not be, if it once was, he said.

Now when I am treating, I can really feel my hands as an embryo. I can feel the wholeness and oneness of this substance we are made of.

It is so beautiful!

Beth

TEETHING

Teething is, of course, an ongoing process in children. Sometimes children can become febrile and congested when the teething process gets out of balance and too much stasis occurs.

Sucking on ice is a naturally calming process, as it can reduce inflammation and pain. Some children actually become quite miserable and need osteopathic intervention.

Examination usually reveals that the anterior portion of the upper and middle face is congested. The fluid dynamics are disturbed, so that there is no local response to the Tide in the anterior region of the upper and middle face. There are no congested lymph nodes or other signs of infection, as this is a sterile inflammatory process. These findings confirm your diagnosis as to the cause of the fever and discomfort.

If the remaining Zone B is operating well, then the treatment is to embrace the lesion field (the zone of the loss of fluid drive) and engage the Third Level Stillness.

This treatment works very quickly, because the lesion is very much an interchange problem with the fluids in the area of the growing teeth.

Note: Recall that the middle face seam between the zygomatic and maxillary arches is where the upper dental arch grow centers are located ... this probably accounts for why we find the "lesion field" in this location.

No direct action is necessary.

MAINTAINING A TREATMENT IN CHILDREN

Third Level Stillness as a family.
Shakedown ... peritoneal sac ... fluid to the fluid.
Massage ... toward the center of the Fluid Body using more than 2 millimeters of pressure.
Bathtub ... child lies on parent on its back ... the parent's hands are under the child's back for support. The child is moved side to side in the water until the water moves the child. Then water and child come to rest ... repeat to tolerance.

THE NORMAL CHILD

The following observations in part or in whole can be made of a normal child. Diagnostics can be accomplished by following these guidelines. By noticing the qualities noted here, one will often find a disease process before it completely unfolds. This is the hallmark of osteopathy and preventive medicine. Traditional diagnostics on children are limited and do not "see" problems until it is "too late."

A child that recovers from an illness is not "cured" until these qualities reappear.

Being at Third Level Stillness creates the receptivity to perceive these things.

Transparency: The Imago Dei is visible. Children radiate the Health as if they were translucent. They feel like a "House Under the Sea" suffused by the Tide.

Provokes Self-Remembering in Adults: When a child comes into our presence, it creates a memory of our own Health. We have a recollection of a deep presence behind life. This feeling connects us with different kinds of memory. If this does not happen, find out why ... is the child restrained somehow? ... Look carefully.

Children Are Healers: If a child physically touches you or looks at you with a gaze of intent, you will feel a communion and healing. Often the depth exceeds any that we witness in osteopathic treatment.

Zone B Is Translucent: Children have no Zone A. The presence of even a small area of A is an alarm telling us to look deeper into the cause.

Innocence: A normal child makes no calculation of loss when following the movement of creation ... when the spirit moves, so moves the child.

Free Will: Children have a unified experience of love ... a freedom to respond without reservation. If this is missing, we must find out why ... it is very important to the child's growth and health.

An Awareness of Belonging to God: There is a good overview of this in *The Spiritual Life of Children* by Robert Coles. If you are not aware of this quality in children, then I recommend the book.

Children Feel the Movement of Creation: This language comes from Phase Eight. It means that a child feels the movement of eternity, somatically. As adults, we very rarely feel this. It is the "now" that mystics like Eckhart Tolle speak about. Creation did not end. It continues.

Children Are a Wholeness: This is a fact that diagnostics can overlook. The growth of a child is done as a whole, not in parts. There is only one fulcrum for the expression of involuntary motion (i.e., growth, primary and secondary respiration).

Children Are Wise: Again, if this is unfamiliar to you, read the book by Robert Coles.

If the above qualities fade or are missing, find the cause.

Live in the Unfolding of the New: There are several points to observe here. First, a child is not aware of the next new quality to arise, and yet they step into it fearlessly. They adapt and begin to sense this new quality with joy. Adults are not even looking for change. Children live on the limit of their understanding and reach for more every day. Adults rarely exceed their limits. A child explores the unfoldment with passion. A child also looks for the source of the "newness" ... they will search and find the fulcrum. Once a normal child finds a garden hose and plays with it a short time ... they will find the faucet and make the connection. This is rapid in a normal child. The exploration is driven by the Intelligence of the Whole, unfolding.

A Normal Child Has Unconditional Love.

One Breath: Normally the Primary and Thoracic Respiration are one with movement of the Whole.

A Divine Gaze: A normal child will look "far away" and stop, filling with Holiness. When they look at you, you may feel the same.

Connected to Third Level Stillness: When adults in the immediate environs are consciously awake to Third Level Stillness, a normal child will respond. A recent report I received on a case highlighted the importance of this. A severely ill child was not responding to treatment as we expected from what the Tide was showing. The clinician made a house call, taught the family about Third Level Stillness, and the response to treatment was greatly accelerated! This fact is food for children.

Rest: Children rest. This is a key quality. If it is missing, find the cause.

Suffering Is Suffused with Love: When children are sick, they do not separate from the Health. Very ill children are still porous to the Health.

Charitable: Children often give away their "best" possessions.

Children Are Direct: The end is the end.

A Normal Child Loves Animals.

Faith: A normal child is comfortable with Mystery.

Imagination: A child should be imagining. Psychologists often think that imagination is a fantasy. It is not. Again, please read Dr. Cole's book. Imagination was recognized by Dr. Sutherland as an asset for adults in understanding Primary Respiration. The word "imagination" originally identified the "highest form of intellect." Today it is a word misused and dead to its real meaning. The art of daydreaming is lost.

Joy

Playfulness

Oneness with All Children

These are qualities to observe in a child to see if they are "normal" from a functional osteopathic model. If any of these are missing ... find out why ... look for the cause ... before they develop a real, serious liability.

"Our skill is proportionate to our understanding of normal." … Dr. Still has directed us to be noble in our discovery of what is normal, what it is like to be normal … and children can help us a great deal.

THE MOTION OF CREATION

Practical

Place the attention outside and inside … two different places …

Sense a third principle flowing through both, without any separation.

During treatment the attention should be moved by the Tide, not by our intention.

Listening

Neutrality

The Newborn's Head

Redemptive Healing and Children

Go Outside

Listen as Far Away as You Can …

Thoracic and Primary Respiration as One

The Motion of Creation

PERCEPTION

Pediatrics from a biodynamic perspective is about a transmutation of the clinician's perception as an observer. This allows the refinement of the sensorium by the "beingness" of the Health in the child.

The Meeting Place is not where we meet the child, but rather where we are met and transmuted by the Health in the child. This is not as easy as one may think, because liking and engaging the child as a friend is a playful and wonderful event, but it does not carry the same sense of elevation and the humbling effect of being on Holy ground and being converted into a witness of incarnating creation and love. It takes a neutral mind to really enter this event, and loving a child is not what I am proposing ... I am saying that we need to be aware that as we are, we are inhibiting the full potential of the indwelling therapeutic process.

Please take the time to start over, again and again, until you feel the somatic sensation of eternity touching you, and watch what your observer does as this happens.

Rebalancing, as you know, is very powerful. We must remember that the stillness in the broken Zone B is the Health, and we must gain the mental agility to ask: Is there a deeper stillness than the one I am in relationship with? ... Watch out for easy access to stillness, as one can miss the deeper and richer potencies (love).

NEUTRALITY

I would like to say a little about neutrality in oneself and how important it is to "being" in relationship with the Health in ourselves, others, and especially children.

Neutral, as Sutherland talked about it, was an automotive metaphor. When a car is in neutral, it is not engaged in any direction ... forward or reverse ... it just sits idling with the engine running. In the ancient teachings, the metaphor about neutrality builds around oneself as a passenger, not the driver.

The driver is the master ... the car is our soma ... the direction of the car is Divine intention ... the journey is a mystery ... rarely do we know exactly where the car is going ... so we remain neutral even when activity begins. The hand of God moves the levers and the gears of the "mechanism" ... giving a sense of ease to the passenger in the car, who is in reality a guest, well served by the master. We do not take the wheel!

A mystic once said, "We should be blank." No anticipation, no plan, no understanding of "whither we go." I like this, but there is fire in the room; one is not blank of senses, only of will.

Neutral is a special room inside the "House Under the Sea" ... the room has no sense of humanity in it, either yours or others'. What is in the Neutral is purity, transparency, and a sweet soft inaudible joy that never leaves the heart to enter the world.

Neutral is a place where one can be free. It is a place where insult and injury are so meaningless that in their presence the joy increases. How strange this seems to our logic. The same energy that hurts the ego adds potency to the spirit when one is neutral. What could wound us heals us.

Neutral is a holistic awareness. It is not "mine." There is no sense of my neutral.

No one can see you unless they are with the Whole, so the projections flow, but the energy never comes in the room ... one is safe from one's ego as well as that of others.

It seems that Dr. Sutherland's affinity with neutral grew from Dr. Still and his colleagues ... I feel from reading Sutherland that he was clearly taken in the Direction of Ease by Still's guiding hand, but then needed to go more directly until he matured (see *Contributions of Thought* and study Sutherland's perceptual odyssey).

The history of the idea of neutral is as old as the oldest recorded history of man's quest for Wholeness (the Vedas), and as old as oral history (the African Bushmen). It is a state of pure nonviolence and charity.

The three forces of Yogic background are emblematic of the three states of Divine expression and are studied in oneself as a tool for approaching a union with God ...

In the Bhagavad Gita there is a battle between the positive and negative forces, but the master takes the student into the space between the duality to begin his teaching ... this is neutral ground.

The images of three forces—active, passive, and neutral—are not to be confused with the three natures of Oneness, where each force is a Divine aspect ... we see this in the Christian Trinity where the three are all perfect and are not active, passive, or neutral but beyond the duality of life that contains "good and evil" that can only be seen clearly in oneself once neutrality is understood as a place of meeting the hope of Wholeness and feeling oneself without the contrast between the three forces of active, passive, and neutral.

Neutrality is the place of rest, repose, and recovery ... it is homeostatic ... transparent to the Seer, so one never feels like the doer or the seer ... one never feels "seen" ... but rather one feels created, as an event on the screen of life, painted by the silent hand of compassion ... one feels made with every other movement in the landscape of the moment, nothing being intrinsically good or evil.

Everything moves with ease, even in the suffering and the lesion, because the neutrality is not positioned in either.

Neutral is so different in a child than in an adult that one may miss it, literally not feel it ... I called it the Desert Neutral after the great teachers who took to the desert to become whole and internally rarefied in their neutrality, i.e., their transparency to Love.

Neutral with indwelling neutrality is suffused with Third Level Stillness.

This is a Meeting Place of all incarnate life.

Therapeutics pass into the neutral substance and a mystery unfolds as the Breath of Divine Love cascades as a therapeutic force across a night desert landscape, filling and leaving behind no visible effects ... only the emptiness of Holy stillness ... healing the physician's sense of limits ... leaving one aware of one's blindness and coarseness ... suffused.

This practical is hard to do on adults, but let's try to learn more about neutrality and the gift of it.

Neutral is the ebb ... where motions subside before a new beginning appears. Neutral is not a means to an end ... it is the end itself.

AT THE CENTER OF OUR BEING

In *Conjectures of a Guilty Bystander* (1966), Thomas Merton writes:

> At the center of our being is a point of nothingness which is untouched by sin and by illusion, a point of pure truth, a point or spark which belongs entirely to God, which is never at our disposal, from which God disposes of our lives, which is inaccessible to the fantasies of our own mind or the brutalities of our own will. This little point of nothingness and of absolute poverty is the pure glory of God in us. It is so to speak his name written in us, as our poverty, as our indigence, as our dependence, as our sonship. It is like a pure diamond, blazing with the invisible light of heaven. It is in everybody, and if we could see it we would see these billions of points of light coming together in the face and blaze of a sun that would make all the darkness and cruelty of life vanish completely . . . I have no program for this seeing. It is only given. But the gate of heaven is everywhere.

DIAGNOSTICS OF THE NEWBORN AND THE INFANT HEAD

Molding, Caput Succedaneum, and Cephalohematoma

Differential diagnosis of these three cranial deformities is important.

Molding of the head is normal, as the cranium folds during labor. It is a phenomenon that is most easily appreciated by bony overlap ... without treatment, it resolves in 72 hours.

Any delay means the fluid drive and potency of the Fluid Body are inadequate to reshape the cranium. The whole of Zone B must be evaluated and treated, if not normal ... when the Whole functions, the cranium will reshape.

Caput succedaneum is a pressure injury only to the scalp. It is not serious, but it may hide a cephalohematoma, which requires more attention. Normal pressure on the head, at the cervical os, and in the vaginal canal cause this edema to occur. Vacuum extractions always cause this, but they may also cause deeper damage inside the periosteal sac. The deeper injury is a bleeding into the periosteal sac that does not leave the sac (i.e., cross the sutures). The distinction between the caput succedaneum and the cephalohematoma is made by palpation. The caput is in the scalp, so the hematoma crosses the sutural lines, whereas with cephalohematoma, the hematoma is in the bone and will not cross sutural lines.

Another possible injury is an epidural bleed into the epidural space under the bone. It cannot be appreciated by palpation, but if one can evaluate the motion in the sacs, it can be sensed. This is more serious and needs consultation if suspected.

Subdural hematoma and deeper traumas are neurologically evident and need consultation. Knowing the layers of the developing head is useful in these and many other situations ... we will review these developmental pathways in our study of the diagnostics of the head.

OSTEOPATHIC THINKING AND THE TREATMENT OF CHILDREN

Dr. Still's writings are not arranged in a textbook and so one must search and reread his words many times. Why do this? Because every time I reread him, my clinical results improve. Just as important, I better understand why he and we need a separate profession from the mainstream of Western medicine.

In *Philosophy of Osteopathy*, he writes about the basic principles he uses in "thinking osteopathy." He was not a structuralist, by his own admission. He considered the whole patient a living reality and sought to establish that wholeness. His vision was that when wholeness was present, all the fluids were free and in abundance. In this state a patient would heal without drugs or remedies other than God's built-in drugstore. The state of disease was, in his mind, the outcome of stasis, fermentation, and putrefaction. Once the "withering field" was refreshed, the patient would heal. Dr. Still's success rate in treating infectious disease made him well respected and sought after as a clinician.

"Think Osteopathy rather than thinking Osteopathically" are the words Sutherland chose to highlight the two different streams of thought in our culture. I will not belabor this point. It is, however, crucial to understanding children and interacting with them.

Sutherland also calls upon us to use our imagination with a capital *I*.

Osteopathic thinking is not what most osteopaths do.

Osteopathic thinking, as described by our founder and his intimate followers, is divergent thinking. It is thinking independently of what one knows. One thinks with an empty mind. There is no cause that is arrived at reductionistically. Cause is met with thinking, knowing, and feeling hands that are connected not to a textbook but to the Health of the patient, and a history directed away from the allopathic ideas and toward the Whole and its moment of compromise.

"Thinking osteopathy" is a science of divergence ... thinking away from the known and into the movement of the unknown, bringing it into the foreground for a moment and letting it pass. This kind of activity is directed toward the whole patient, not the cause of the symptoms. It embraces stillness in the center of the process.

There are books on this subject. Or you can watch children! Intelligence is not really about a graduate education.

Convergent thinking is the norm for adults. It is thinking that moves toward a predetermined goal, that is set in the reduction of data into a format, or a belief, or bias. Convergent thinking is closed before it starts. It fears imagination. It is dependent on the known facts. It is not reason. It is not imagination. Both reason and imagination are higher functions. Still saw reason as a Divine wisdom, a gift ... as did Aristotle.

Divergent thinking moves away from any predetermined goal. It is open to the "not yet" that is coming in the moment of being. It is not afraid of inadequacies or failure, nor is it bold. It is open and not reductionistic. It is creative within the movements of life, not one's past knowledge. Unlike convergence, it is patient, neutral, and does not lead the patient or jump to conclusions. It sees the whole.

This process includes diagnosis and history, brought to a point of meaningfulness by the Health in both parties. It is often curative, as it happens. The chief complaint is a doorway into a story of how the functional reserve in the whole became compromised. The parts follow a larger picture; they do not lead it.

This is how it is with children ...

Children can really help us undo our convergence. But we must meet them on their own landscape.

And with adults like Drs. Still, Sutherland, Wales, Becker, Day, Laughlin, Johnston, et cetera.

Recommended Reading

Philosophy of Osteopathy, Andrew Taylor Still D.O.... it is a small book; how does he want us to think?

"The Tour of the Minnow" ... last article in *Contributions of Thought,* William Garner Sutherland D.O.

Oxford English Dictionary, Unabridged ... see definition for "imagination"

The Spiritual Life of Children, Robert Coles

Sir Ken Robinson, YouTube.com, several videos with great discussions on children and divergent thinking

CHILDREN AS ONE

We have spoken about many things relating to children that are very universal and beautiful … there is more.

Children can move the therapeutic forces in a direction that reflects great compassion flowing through them, without any spiritual "training."

They are natural saints, or angels, bringing validation to an open heart.

It seems that as one explores their world, one comes to a sense that each child universally sees all children as a single appendage of creation.

One can explore this easily by adding this dimension to the space of the treatment.

Also, there is a redemptive spirit in them that allows for the treatment to go to others in need … this is not uncommon. Redemptive prayer is practiced in most traditions … it is prayer that is done for others, like fasting for others, or doing penance for others. Gandhi was well known for this kind of "work."

The Wholeness of a child's heart is beyond what we can imagine.

BREATHING IN CHILDREN AND ADULTS

Our sense of breathing, as a function in the cranial field of osteopathy, has always been that there are three basic breaths: Thoracic or Secondary Respiration, Primary Respiration, and the Breath of Life.

Thoracic respiration is a metabolic event that begins at conception and is not a mechanical but rather a physiological event. It is much more than the diaphragm, the lungs, and the ribs. It is intracellular metabolic fire, it heats us, and, as we shall see, it has therapeutic power. Sutherland began his journey appreciating much more about thoracic respiration than we commonly teach. His choice of the fourth ventricle for a CV4 was because his goal in treatment was to bring the motion of thoracic respiration to a highly refined neutral, where the breathing was almost still. He saw this neutral of thoracic respiration as a primary indicator that the fluids, especially the lymphatics, were free to find homeostasis. Rereading his comments is inspiring. In children we have discovered that thoracic respiration has transmutative therapeutic potency.

Primary Respiration is hallmarked by an inhalation period and exhalation period (Sutherland). Primary Respiration has a variety of rates. The common rates are two to three cycles per minute and 100 seconds per cycle.

In the two-to-three-cycle-per-minute rate, the period of inhalation and the period of exhalation each last one second ... the whole cycle being 24 seconds or two and a half cycles per minute.

The rate of the Long-Tide is 50 seconds for the exhalation period and 50 seconds for the inhalation period, the whole cycle being 100 seconds (Becker).

The Cranial Rhythmic Impulse is not considered a rate because it is the same as thoracic respiration and is highly variable ... it is considered by many to be a nontherapeutic rate. This view is not appreciated by everyone and needs your personal exploration as to its validity.

As you may recall, during therapeutics in adults, the inhalation phase is prolonged and the exhalation phase is silent. This phenomenon demonstrates that rates are not present while transmutation is occurring. That when the treatment period is ending, there comes a Stillpoint that heralds the coming of a new neutral. The stillpoint is the height of the transmutative period and is followed by neutral at a deeper level than the beginning neutral. The rate also slows, so that the initial neutral is often breathing faster than the neutral at the end point after transmutation occurs.

This change to a slower rate indicates a greater wholeness, a deeper neutral that is more stable, and greater therapeutic outcomes.

Eventually, we come to a neutral with no rate ... just a steady Dynamic Stillness that hovers in the fluid indefinitely.

Our first practical is about reuniting the Wholeness of breathing.

When a child has surgery, very often they separate Thoracic Respiration from the one fulcrum that it previously shared with "all the breath." The chief symptom of this is often a perceptual change in the child, one of distance ... look into their eyes and you will see they feel "lost," separated from the Wholeness; they become confused and "clingy."

Often a simple resynchronization of thoracic respiration, easily done, produces immediate and lasting perceptual shifts. In my own practice, I was missing this easy diagnosis because I assumed that thoracic and Primary Respiration were separate functions, with separate potencies and fulcrums ... this is not true in children.

Now I am wondering how many autistic and perceptually fragile children are missing this linkage, and I wonder if we are treating in too complex a manner in some cases ... I recommend that in perceptually challenged children, you explore this benefit of resynchronization through the diaphragm, and see if it sorts out some of the dilemmas that we face.

THE POTENCY AND SUFFUSION OF ZONE B BY THORACIC RESPIRATION

Practical

In children you will find, upon close evaluation, that thoracic respiration is as potent a healing force as Primary Respiration is in adults ... !

We can revisit Thoracic Respiration and Zone B in adults and explore this terrain that is so different in children and adults.

With your hands on the posterior midline of the diaphragm, synchronize with the breathing and watch the whole patient ... what transpires?

Children treat faster and more easily, as adults usually have a split in their fulcrum.

THORACIC RESPIRATION AND PRIMARY RESPIRATION IN CHILDREN

Thoracic and Primary Respiration begin at or before conception. They move as one branch of a tree—one fulcrum, two rates.

Watch the leaves and branches of a tree in the breeze, and you will see what I mean.

When children lesion, they lesion as a whole, and often this relationship, this oneness of breathing, remains. So we check for this; hopefully it is as it should be.

If the breaths are separate, they should resynchronize as the whole of Zone B becomes neutral. This can be appreciated easily. As the Thoracic Respiration moves into a deep inhalation (big sigh), the Primary Respiration also makes a big inhalation. This augmentation is automatic.

If this does not occur when Primary Respiration rebalances and swells, then have the child breathe in at the same moment as the Tide swells. This will resynchronize the system. If not, note that it is important (this principle was used by Sutherland and is called breath augmentation). This helps Zone A and Zone B reunite as one movement in which A transmutes.

A BRIEF DISCUSSION OF THE ANTERIOR FONTANEL

This fontanel is remarkably interesting. It lies on the central sagittal seam. The closure of the fontanel takes many changes to accomplish.

It is diamond-shaped, and the angles close before the central axis of the fontanels. The posterior diamond closes before the anterior portion does.

After molding recedes at three days post natal, the diamond should be symmetrical. If not, treat the Fluid Body, and watch for symmetry to appear ... early closure or asymmetry can be addressed only early on.

If one is meticulous and watches carefully, small distortions reflect the whole. Cause can be anywhere, not just locally. So we treat the whole.

After the molding ends and the symmetry is restored, the four recesses of the diamond have their own story to tell ... each one at a different tempo. For example, anteriorly, the lateral angle tends to elevate above the fontanel, then recedes to be on the same plane as the fontanel. This is because the brain grows quickly here; the fluid field elevates as the new inner layer is created. Once the old superficial layer is reabsorbed, the bone again feels level with the tissue. This only happens early in growth, and not as the growth of the bones gains physiological momentum. So ... do not think that there is a superior vertical strain when this happens!

If we look at the lateral view of the infant head, we can see a downward slope to the area in front of the coronal suture. This is the anterior dural girdle fluid field. It is often misdiagnosed as an inferior vertical strain. As I stated above, as the frontal fluid fields expand, the bone thickens from the outside as the inner layer is reabsorbed ... when this happens in the first months, it feels like a superior vertical strain ... close observation will tell you it is bony growth, and that the inner layer is being absorbed as the outer layer increases. The downward slope disappears during this time and lessens as the frontal area grows. This does not narrow the lateral angles of the fontanel. This is how we can be sure of our findings. Palpation of the anterior dural girdle is possible for several years.

As we watch the fontanel change, there are changes throughout the whole central sagittal seam.

The lower sternum follows the anterior fontanel ... it closes from above downward ... this can easily be palpated and followed along with the changes above ... one seam is closing throughout the body. This helps us to be aware of healthy activity and to pick up changes in growth dynamics early, which makes treatments more effective and preventative.

The lateral sides of the fontanels close, then the posterior, and then the anterior portion of the fontanel. Closure of lambda is much earlier. We can sense a continuity along the anterior midline (not the seam): two frontals, two nasal, two vomer plates, two sides of the hyoid, two sides of the sternum from above then downward (same time as anterior fontanel), the navel is often "open" for several months and closes within the first year, and so on to the feet. A study of this is not in any book, but you can follow your children and find these truths helpful. The neural and visceral tissues are moving toward center as well.

Another note that is helpful here: If you follow the lateral angles of the fontanel in an infant, you will come to the coronal suture, then to the anterior inferior fontanel, then you can go anterior along the zygomatic suture to the orbit and travel through the fissure, back to the root of the sphenoid, and directly above is the fontanel ... giving you a feel for the whole anterior cranial fossa.

The vertical line from the bregma to the tip of the notochord (junction of pre-post sphenoid) is used for orientation in treating Down syndrome.

Note: there is a horizontal line from the tip of the notochord to the anterior inferior fontanel.

There are diagonal lines through the bosses to the tip of the notochord.

There is a diagonal line from lambda to the tip of the notochord.

We can explore these craniometrics and the sagittal seam in a practical.

We will check the seam and exchange our findings. Then treat.

THE SAGITTAL SEAM

The idea of seams is from the Biodynamics Phases and does not appear in any other book. The word "seam" is used to denote a fold that occurs early in the movement of the whole embryo, as it begins to define form and spaces for growth. We see this early when the "seam" between the thoracic and abdomen cavities appears, with the descent of the diaphragm/heart/lungs and creation of the foregut. The seams precede the segments and the functions. The segments are oriented to the notochords while seams are formed as the whole moves around an invisible midline. The seams are related to the Dynamic Stillness of the central midline and treat easily at that level of potency.

The seams of the development of the head and upper cervical region are discussed in Phase Five. This knowledge is of great help in treating children, and especially children with Down syndrome. Today, we will look at the central sagittal seam in the whole patient. Down syndrome will be addressed later.

The central sagittal seam in the infant head creates the space of orientation for the alignment and growth of the layers we explored earlier in the course. Imagine a seam before there is any brain, dura, bones, etc. The seam appears in a functionally empty house filled with protoplasm. As the protoplasm becomes "something" it aligns with the seams, which, I believe, contain the pattern being unfolded and the tempo of that process.

To follow this line of visualization, follow the seam from the sagittal suture into the interior. You will find the two sides of the falx that develop along the seam and move toward the seam as they grow inward from the periphery.

If we go deeper, we find the central fissure of the brain. Again, this appears before the tissue around it and guides the unfoldment toward it.

If we go deeper still, we come to the two thalamic nuclei, the central fulcrum of the third ventricle, and the two sides of the third ventricle from which the two eyes emerge and grow into the orbital region.

The lamina terminalis and optic chasm are on the seam.

The seam traverses the whole body as a central sagittal seam.

A place of orientation for the two halves of the body.

Perhaps a place of continued origin of new cellular material.

It functions as one seam and is not an effect of the surrounding tissues.

It lesions as one place throughout the whole being.

THE NAVAJO BASKET

Our research into the anterior fontanel has led us in many directions. None of these directions included reading books.

One task was to observe the changes in the anterior fontanel as the first year of life progressed. How does the pattern of the fontanel shift, and when? ... No books were used. We simply watched our patients.

We will discuss this later.

My family and I were driving through the Grand Canyon area of the US when we came upon some Navajo Native Americans. They were selling their crafts. A young Navajo, about 22, saw my son Sam and gave him a turquoise stone to carry with him through his life. We began to speak.

My fellow traveler was a Navajo who cherished his tradition and oral teaching.

He was, at first, speaking about the migration of his people from Mongolia to the southwest of North America, a journey that began as much as 20,000 years ago.

In 20,000 years one thing has remained unmovable ... the oral teaching about life and a sacred map to Wholeness ...

This gentle young man wanted to speak about the story that is carried in the weaving of the Navajo basket.

The basket begins with the hole at the top ... the soft spot on a child's head ... this is the place where the love, and the teaching, and the power of the community pass into the child ... it is the doorway through which "learning" occurs on the journey of life. The weaving in the basket is based upon the labyrinth of a life's journey that we all travel ... at times our lessons are learned quickly and we come back to the center over a shorter path ... sometimes the length of the lesson is longer, and it takes us more time to come back to the center and gain wisdom; so reports the image in the weaving.

Coming back to the hole, the emptiness at the center, there is a turning of the lesson into wisdom ... some lessons take a lifetime before the path of self-knowledge leads to a return to the self and the love and the wisdom and power ... at the emptiness of the hole (anterior fontanel).

When a child begins to laugh from the center, usually after walking for a while, then the weaving of the journey of life begins.

When the child starts laughing at life, with life, and at himself ... then there is a celebration in the tribe because the child has begun the journey ... the child fills a woven basket with salt ... and as the visitors come to celebrate ... the child hands out salt from the basket to each person. Giving the most precious and valued food, salt ... celebrating by giving the best you have away to those who come to celebrate your "birthday" ... giving the best from the center of the basket ... reaching in and handing it to others to benefit from ... charity begins the path, it is the first step.

The story struck me deeply ... especially when he said that the stories had died and were coming back, even in the schools.

As we both "sighed," a great silence filled the air. I asked if I could look closely at a basket.

He said sadly, "There are none, there has been a 13-year drought and the sycamores are not growing." Another pause filled with respect and reverence for Great Spirit ... then we spoke some more.

"You know," he said ... "It takes many hours and materials to make a basket. The design is our story. Nowadays, people take the design and make cheap baskets in Pakistan, then sell them as Navajo baskets for twenty dollars." ... A sadness came over me ... I waited through it ... he was still ... I read his silence as neutrality.

The story helped me a great deal to see that my complaints about people stealing osteopathy and cheapening our oral tradition had angered me, and here was a young man who saw his losses as Divine will ... An old wound began to soften and drain ... the incision was painless; a wound that felt so deep became a part of communion with the weaver of life. His story and behavior had healed me.

The hole at the top of the basket (and a child's head) ... is there so the weaver can pattern a lifetime that begins with laughter and charity ... the hole creates the basket ... its form and its meaning.

As you watch children at play, or during treatment, you may see a ribbon of grace flowing into the child and filling the Desert Neutral. It flows through the top ... just like the Navajo story relates.

If you have not seen this ... just watch ... you will.

IT IS NOT POSSIBLE TO FIND ANY AXIAL LESION IN THE SKULL

Axial lesions are lesions occurring at the sphenobasilar synchondrosis. The idea, as you know, is that lesions are modulated by the reciprocal tension membrane around or through a midline that traverses the sphenobasilar symphysis articulation. The lesions are called by names like side bending, torsion, vertical strain, lateral strain, etc. They are parallels to the vertebral body lesions.

Axial motion is an outdated model. There is much more than biomechanics going on in a living system. It is a breathing, transmuting metabolic event that we sense as motion.

The lesioning process occurs in the whole physiological unit, not just in structure. The foundation of form is not structural; it is a living physiological event that is constantly replacing the old with the new—if we are Health, i.e., expressing the capacity for neutral. The form of something is its functional nature. Structure is a bad term because it is static, whereas the form is being renewed constantly.

This means the old must be transformed and a new form expressed … this is the basis for growth and development in children. It occurs so fast that there is no function that is static, i.e., structural. In the process described above, the geometry and position of function and form is from protoplasm into the metabolic fields by biodynamic/biokinetic forces that are not organized by the central nervous system but by what we call the Fluid Body. Consider the fact that the repositioning of tissue is a function of neutral and the Fluid Body. This is not to say that the intrinsic spinal muscles cannot hold a lesion and, if de-facilitated, cannot "reposition" because the muscle tone has changed. This lesioning process is not segmental. It just appears that way. Cause is in the whole organism as a unit. This includes psychological and physiological aberrancies in the lesioning process. Osteopathic is different from allopathic. Cause for us is not local.

When the fluid fields lesion, the fluid distorts. The distortion is not reducible without a Neutral. The fluid holds it and the tissues take on the form.

The remolding of the head after birth; the movement of the teeth and their position, which begins at six weeks in utero and continues throughout life; the renewal of scar tissue, which requires the old to be transmuted and the new form to appear—these are all metabolic events, not structural.

Zone B is the Fluid Body that lesions. At neutral, the Fluid Body is directed toward normal by the therapeutic forces of the Health.

"It's the not-yet in the now, the taste of the fruit that does not-yet exist, hanging the blossom on the bough."

Laurens van der Post, Venture to the Interior, (1979).

THE TASTE OF THE FRUIT

We assume cause and effect, but deductive reasoning in treatment has no value in realizing the whole, which is already complete at conception. What is happening is that time (the ego's fear of death) veils eternity. We believe that eternity is not here ... it *is* here, and the Health exists in it and is transparent to it.

Cause and effect, as we summate clinically, is a lesion coming from our ego and not from our Health ... it is an illusion. We treat the illusion, and the illusion operates somewhere else.

What appears to be the "not yet" is fully here now. The "not yet" is the taste of the fruit hanging the blossom on the tree ... growth proceeds from the end of the future, in the now of eternity. It is done. We believe it is linear and sequential. Where is the power and where is the timing? ... It is the fruit that is moving the whole toward the known, not the unknown.

Look at how you analyze yourself and your attributes ... and others. We think we know "cause and effect" in others and ourselves. So-and-so is behaving that way because of ... ? This is not the whole picture. Can you taste the fruit? If not, you will certainly harm yourself and others by your belief that your analysis is correct ... then you are upset and determined to treat it or be heartbroken ... Find the taste of the fruit that hangs the blossom ... see it in yourself and others, then you will feel a different world ... like a child. Then you can let eternity pass through you, as it does a child, and you will transmit, not produce, love.

Children do not analyze themselves ... but they do feel the fruit and by its taste they are joy.

Adults prune the fruit from their senses, then believe that someone else pruned the tree. Then they make up a journey to grow the fruit ...

all this is a lesion and exhaustion and is not happening. The fruit is fully present. What good does it do to try to become what has already happened? Or to treat a child's lesion rather than tasting the fruit and the whole finished product?

Why would Dr. Wales say, "When the acute lesion is gone, osteopathy begins, and that's when we treat the patient"?

Gone from our minds as soon as possible is better.

Practical

Find the taste of the fruit in the patient,

without deduction…

help your senses remember the end of the future,

which is conception.

The Taste of Wholeness

The Constant Motion Toward Normal

BIODYNAMICS OF OSTEOPATHY BOOK SERIES

This book is one of a series of twelve *Biodynamics of Osteopathy* books. It is recommended that you read the whole series in order, as each book builds on the understanding from prior books. It is also recommended that you seek experienced teachers and mentors to help you experience the full depth of the information given.

The full series is as follows:

Phase One is about involuntary motion, which is motion present in the whole and in the lesion. We learn to synchronize with the breathing of Primary Respiration before we approach any treatment. This synchronization is the key to working with stable rates and not irritating the system. The principle of synchronizing with a healthy aspect of the patient suffuses the whole teaching program. This synchronization shifts our awareness to a different level of receptivity, which allows us to see Primary Respiration rather than the lesion field, and this eventually leads us to an understanding of the intention of Primary Respiration.

Phase Two is about communication with the natural laws of healing that surround activity at 2 to 3 cycles per minute. We synchronize with the breathing of Primary Respiration and also add the skill of sensing the fulcrum, the Stillness through which the breathing creates form and function. It is a different kind of synchronization from that in Phase One, shifting our awareness more deeply. As this occurs, the treatment automatically expresses itself. The end point of treatment, when compared with Phase One, reveals several differences. We find this kind of synchronization works exclusively with the fluid body and the outcome of treatment is more complete than when working with tissue alone.

Phase Three is centered around the activities of the Long Tide (100 second cycle). We explore an indwelling therapeutic force already present in the lesion field. We learn that the dural system is not made-up of three sickles but rather a series of folds in a sac, arising during growth and development. We see the relationship between the upper and lower dural sacs, awakening us to the independence of two separate tentorium cerebelli. We discover that zone D, the horizon, and the Wire (along which the Long Tide moves during its intended therapeutic course) are all linked as natural laws pertaining to this level of Primary Respiration.

Phase Four focuses on the Midline, a place where the spatial relationships are expressed as a whole. It synchronizes and centers us in such a way that we become aware of Zone D and the Dynamic Stillness. The Third Level Stillness in Phase Four is different from the Stillness in the other Phases – we are centered by the Stillness at the center of creation. Our intention is replaced by the intention of the Tide which can facilitate our spiritual path.

Phase Five is about *the face*. As we approach the face, we use all of the principles that we have learned in Phase One, Two, Three, and Four. We work with automatic shifting and notice differences from how the face is viewed by older models within Osteopathy in the Cranial Field. As we synchronize with the therapeutic presence of the Long Tide we see what we can learn about the face from that landscape. We also work with Seams, Dynamic Stillness, and Ignition.

Phase Six is a continuation of our journey into the Wholeness that generates life and delivers therapeutic forces that transmute lesions once Neutral is expressed. It is a mixture of activities centered around the outside presence of Primary Respiration as something that is a non-biological force and that has a persona. We will also continue to explore seams and then move on to the extremities, first in the embryological terms and then as Sutherland taught them in his work called PowerPoints. Phase 6 is a time to build your understanding of the Tide and refine your skills.

Phase Seven highlights the Health. Dr. Still's famous comment "Find the Health; anyone can find disease," has plagued many minds over the last century. We come to the clear vision of several indwelling aspects of the Health: Love ... liquid light ... and a diamond matrix. A approach to the terminally ill and dying patient is addressed. In the somatic sensation of the Tide passing through the House Under the Sea, our awareness is transmuted by the Health. The lesion is seen as a precognitive act of the Health. Thoracic Respiration, Primary Respiration, and Ignition are as One. The landscape is vast ... and the principles of healing are even more substantial than we have previously experienced..

Phase Eight is a deeper exploration of seams, balanced rhythmic interchange, and the Flame of Intention as a therapeutic modality. Phase Eight is the culmination of our awareness of Wholeness, and ultimately brings us to the Divine Presence, Unconditional Love and Oneness. The living Tide dominates the awareness while forms move to the background. One feels the Breath of Creation in oneself as the Center of Wholeness. One feels the Unfoldment of oneself as one is Created. Our consciousness is a gift; we do not own it and if we try to control it we lose Wholeness.

Phase Nine is when we are able to fully evaluate and treat the Central Nervous System and the Eye. We also address Fire and the therapeutic modality of the Shakedown. True action is moved from Love and makes our perception exist. This Love is self-emptying and by its nature allows us to Serve as part of the Perfect. Perception can be used to Serve something other than ourselves. We have attempted to enter this balance point between the Perfect and the Disease ... it is a point where the whole of everything is suspended by Love as it works to incarnate the Complete. In the balance point of everything is The Intention of the Tide following the movement of the distortion back to a True relationship with the Blueprint of Life.

Pediatrics One explores how children grow as a whole, not in parts as we sometimes believe. Children live in the Direction of Ease of motion present in their fluid metabolic fields, otherwise they get uncomfortable and require assistance. Does your treatment directly support the whole, or does it assume to support the whole? We realize children are not adults and cannot be treated as adults are. We approach the therapeutic modality of the "Meeting Place", prenatal and postnatal periods, the treatment of the pelvis during pregnancy, fetal malposition and labor.

Pediatrics Two is where we deepen in the perceptive awareness necessary to approach the treatment of children. We deepen in our appreciation of Wholeness, the three levels of Stillness and the "Meeting Place". We approach "Desert Neutral", where therapeutics pass into the neutral substance, and a mystery unfolds as the breath of Divine love cascades as a therapeutic force across a night desert landscape, filling and leaving behind no visible effects. We further address treatment of the pelvis and the uterus during pregnancy. We explore thoracic and Primary Respiration in children, and the Family Circle.

Pediatrics Three is where we continue to study the therapeutic Flow of Attention. We deepen in Third Level Stillness and the Meeting Place. The Meeting Place is easily misinterpreted ... our observer must be so still and neutral that the process can be seen as it happens. The central nervous system in the child can be finally approached for evaluation and treatment. We explore teething and also the "locked up head". We use the therapeutic modality of the Flame of Intention, and its connection to the Breath of Life. Everything is transparent to the Breath of Life.

ABOUT THE AUTHOR

James Jealous, D.O. (1943–2021), was an osteopathic physician, teacher, and writer. His life's work was founding and developing **Biodynamics of Osteopathy**, a unique methodology he established within the field of osteopathy, following the lineage of Dr. A.T. Still and Dr. W.G. Sutherland.

He was born in Saco, Maine, and since his father was an osteopathic physician, he was around osteopathy from an early age. He studied at Kirksville College of Osteopathic Medicine in Missouri (now the A.T. Still University of Health Sciences), graduating in 1970. He then set up practice in rural Maine as an osteopathic primary care physician.

Over time, Dr. Jealous saw parallels between the work of embryologist Dr. Erich Blechschmidt and that of osteopathic physician Dr. William Garner Sutherland. This inspiration led him to create his own body of work. In the early 1990s, he began teaching "A Biodynamic View of Osteopathy in the Cranial Field," which, as he developed his specific methodology, was refined to "Biodynamics of Osteopathy."

A deeply spiritual person, he felt most at home in the natural world and was an avid fisherman and hiker.

For more information, please visit:
https://BiodynamicsOfOsteopathy.com

There is a wind passing through ...
it is the motion of creation,
the eternal motion of Divine love.